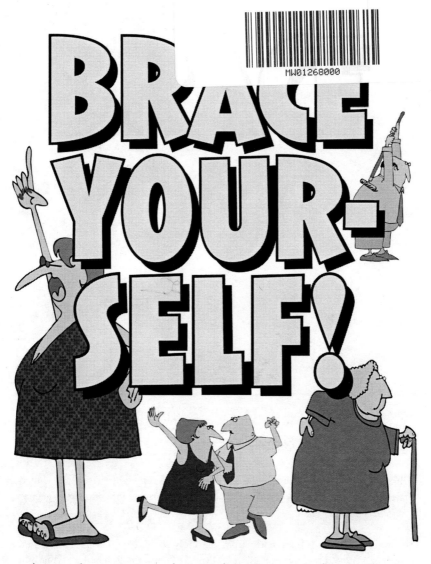

BRACE YOUR-SELF!

An insider's wit & wisdom for living younger than you are

Bee Oldfield

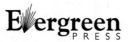

Evergreen
PRESS

Mobile, Alabama

ISBN 978-1-58169-484-0
For Worldwide Distribution
Printed in the U.S.A.
Evergreen Press
P.O. Box 191540 • Mobile, AL 36619
800-367-8203

Contents

Dear Reader-Friend,

Oh, we haven't met, but I call you friend with hopes you'll feel that way after reading my little book.

Brace Yourself! is about what to expect heading toward your 80s and 90s from someone who's been there. As I move down this road, I notice many little things I might have changed earlier had I known what to expect—things that would have made it easier for me now. With the benefit of hindsight and without rehashing standard (though worthwhile) guidance we have all heard about getting old, my goal is to offer practical, down-to-earth tips for making life easier in one's later years. Most of the ideas can be adapted or tinkered with to fit individual circumstances.

In addition to preparation tips, I also will share how it feels and how I cope (as cheerfully as possible) with some of the less desirable aspects of old age. I hope you'll find an idea or two—or maybe just a different way of looking at something—that will work for you.

—*Bee Oldfield*

Introduction

Penned by an unknown author, a verse from an old poem-song begins:

"Oh, I was born ten thousand years ago,
And there really isn't a thing that I don't know."

But wait. Even Methuselah wasn't *that* old, and neither am I, nor is my husband, Charlie. It was only 93 years ago when the two of us came on board, and there are admittedly several things we still don't know. But it occurred to me lately that there may be a few things we have picked up along 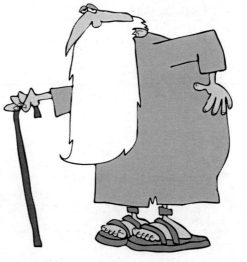 the way to make life in one's 80s and 90s a little easier, if one is warned in advance.

So I asked myself: *How might lessons I've learned be passed along?* Over my many years, folks have fairly often commented, "You should write a book!" The suggestion—though good for a chuckle—drew little attention from me until now. Somehow *now* does seem a good time to take the idea seriously. Competition among us nonagenarian authors should not be a big problem. Maybe I have a helpful suggestion or two, and by my reckoning, it's now or never.

So without further ado, join me as we brace for life beyond 80.

THE BIG "IF"

Before we get down to the nitty-gritty and you start evaluating how some of the suggestions in this book might work for you, let's deal with the big "if."

At this point in our lives, it is unlikely we can do everything we once did. Each of us carries around a personal suitcase of needs, limitations, and unique circumstances. Throughout this book, I'll offer various ideas, trusting you'll look at them through an "If I Can" lens—meaning if you're able to use them. No one expects you to follow a suggestion that requires an ability you no longer have or something you can't afford.

Feel free to pick and choose what might work for you (maybe with a little encouragement from those who love you).

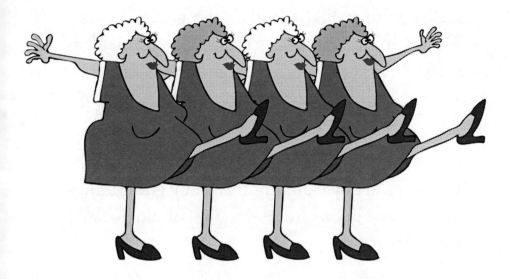

1

WHAT'S IT LIKE
TO BE 93?

More than a quarter of a century ago, popular actress Bette Davis got it right when she said, "Old age ain't no place for sissies."

It really isn't!

Please don't take exception to the phrase "old age." Some folks seem to want to disguise reality with palliatives like "the golden years." To me, even "seniors" strikes me as a shield to hide behind.

I am old. And I'm not ashamed to say it. To my way of thinking, growing old gracefully seems a goal worth embracing. And it seems right to start by claiming the many good things at this time in our lives—in spite of old age and its limitations.

My mother's clear expectation for me when I was young was that I could, and should, wait for a knight in shining armor riding a white horse before I promised my hand in marriage. This almost cost me the good husband I've had these many years because he had neither shining armor nor a white horse! But I saw the twinkle in his eyes that said he was a good man. And he hung in there until I said yes.

Sixty-four years later, we still have each other, we still live in our own home, and we still have most of our own teeth. We both get around under our own steam—no canes, walkers, scooters or such, yet—and Charlie plays golf, mall-walks most days, and still drives our car.

We also enjoy having our two daughters in our hometown. Though very different from each other, both are unquestionably credits to the human race (no prejudice here). We have a small but loving family including four promising, young adult grandchildren, along with assorted other loved ones who might as well be family.

Because we receive help a half day each week from a treasured housekeeper (who, in a way, is more like a third daughter in the care she shows for us), we manage to maintain a reasonably tidy household. We plan, shop for, prepare, and clean up after our meals, and we tend to and enjoy our household pets.

Unfortunately, while I was writing this book, the time came for our almost 16-year-old kitty, Widget, to go. Since then, in the spirit of thinking young, we acquired two very rambunctious kittens, Winnie and Pooh. Cute as they are, I still ask myself: *What were we thinking?* We refer to the two of them as "the demolition crew."

There's little doubt we are ahead of the game compared to many, but let me quickly say: getting old still is not a bed of roses. It is the epitome of the slippery slope.

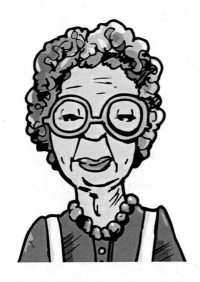

On that momentous day three years ago when I entered my tenth decade, someone flipped a switch—at least that's how it felt to me—and just about everything seemed to come unglued. Friends and family didn't see the sudden change, but boy, did I feel it!

Overnight, the world seemed an unfamiliar place. Until then, every birthday simply added one more year to my age; since turning 90, every birthday increases an "end-times" mindset, reminding me I have one less year to go. This prompts me to do a lot of thinking

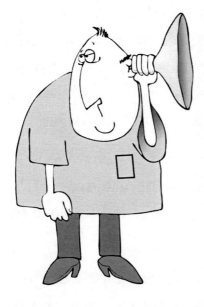

about the hereafter, as in "what did I come in here after?"

With no warning at all, my get-up-and-go got up and went, taking with it most of my eyesight and hearing. Without those senses functioning reasonably well, my equilibrium turned to a fall hunting for a place to happen.

I don't know what went with my sense of smell, but when it left, my sense of taste went too. Not that things taste bad, they just don't taste. "Season to taste" is a thing of my past.

The shakes—"essential tremor" in old-folk talk—took my dexterity. Most of my life I have sewn, crocheted, knitted, painted, etc. My hands have always been busy. Now I can barely replace a button. Even stepping into my house shoes takes on the appearance of a lively River Dance rehearsal!

And then there is the pesky little issue of brain function. Mine still seems fairly dependable, except where even a smidgen of short-term memory is involved. I can't even remember what it was I was trying to forget!

"Almost everything hurts and what doesn't hurt doesn't work" used to be a clever little quip. Now some days it hits a little too close to home to seem funny.

Why am I telling you all this? Just to give you a little of my background, and that's enough of that. By this point most all of us have a lengthy list of woes and, well, we all know recounting them grows tedious. So let's move on, roll up our sleeves, throw back our shoulders, lift our heads high, and get to work. Let's prepare to hang in there, making the best of what lies ahead.

2

FIND YOUR BLESSINGS—
COUNT THEM OFTEN

When my husband was in the market for a
new car a year or so ago, he and our son-in-law
had quite a discussion regarding the merits of a

five-year versus a ten-year extended warranty. Now that's living with optimism!

Charlie is the youngest 93-year-old you are likely to ever meet. He started young saying, "You can get old if you want, but I'm not going to." I'm here to tell you that it worked. His positive attitude, cheerful spirit, and active body keep him younger than many 70-year-olds I know.

Charlie is living proof of Oliver Wendell Holmes' wisdom: "To be 70 [or 90] years young is sometimes far more cheerful and hopeful than to be 40 years old."

Charlie counts his blessings every day. And he reminds me to do the same. Whether by his ever-present, cheerful humming (which admittedly causes me to take off my hearing aids at times) or his jolly laugh, he brings happiness into our household. I try to respond in kind.

Counting one's blessings regularly is a good idea at any age but especially for us oldsters. On a bad day, it may take a conscious effort to stop and look for something good, but if we do, chances are high that we'll find it.

And while we're at it, let's remember the equally important task of expressing thanks to

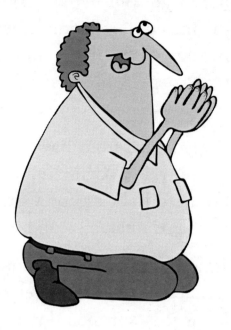

our heavenly Father for every blessing—no matter how hard we have to look for it. Prayer time brings the perfect opportunity for serious reflection, evaluation, and decision making.

My prayers are multi-purpose, but three things I seldom fail to ask for are the strength and ability to stay: 1) useful, 2) cheerful, and 3) a nuisance to no one.

My theology stems from so many denominations that I'm a square peg in a round hole most anywhere I go. But my father's faith was deep enough (including 50 simultaneous years as adult Sunday School teacher and Boy Scoutmaster) to give me a solid religious grounding.

In 1940 I graduated from Baylor University, but since I married Charlie, a lifetime Lutheran, I've tried to be a good Christian first and an acceptable Lutheran second.

Although both of us were born into devoted Christian families, we don't *talk* religion much of the time, but it is our intention to *live* it all the time . . . doing the right things . . . caring about all our neighbors and friends in addition to our family and church family . . . and responding to all in loving, caring ways.

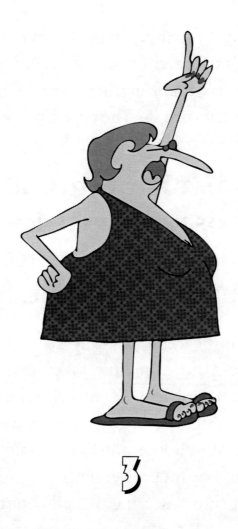

3

HOLD YOUR OWN!

Overriding all others in importance, my first suggestion is this: steel yourself against being hurt when people begin to talk down to you as never before. You may even hear actual baby talk. There's no need to be rude when we resist being patronized, but neither are we required to match the picture of those who view us as being in our second childhood.

DON'T BUY INTO THE IMAGE OF INCOMPETENCE AND CHILDISHNESS WISHED UPON US BY SOME.

If we're not careful, we may even bring it on ourselves. If you let people talk down to you, others watch and leap to the conclusion that you are no longer able to function well. Even more, when we choose not to do something we can still do, we fuel a perception of ourselves we may not find flattering. It's all about image.

Most of us cherish our independence. To preserve it, *act* competent. I'm not advising something artificial. No, this is about holding on to what you've got and showing it. Don't let others do for you what you can (and should) do for yourself.

You also hold your own when you preserve your identity. Many, if not most of us, manage to stay the same inside, at least to ourselves, no matter how many years pile up. We must honor this. Maybe it is a truism worth repeating: in my mind, I'm still the girl I was at 30. Well, okay, maybe 50—even though my body doesn't realize it.

DON'T BE PUSHED INTO BECOMING A STEREOTYPE OF WHAT OTHERS THINK OLD PEOPLE ARE SUPPOSED TO BE!

Someone once said: "Age is all in your mind. The trick is to keep it from creeping down into your body." If we can hold on to the knowledge that we are competent (at least in some areas of our lives), we may manage to retain a fair portion of our self-respect. And that may help us ignore plenty of demeaning juniors.

Health problems, speech problems, and just plain getting around problems may add to the impression we have gone backwards. It be-hooves us to hang in there, holding our own and *remaining the same person* in spite of superficial suggestions otherwise.

Keep an Advocate in the Wings

No matter how competent and independent you are today, the time will come when you catch yourself unexpectedly muddled or confused—perhaps over an interchange with a doctor regarding a health issue, a computer-generated bill with more numbers than paper, or a word processor that does what it wants, not what you tell it to do. This complex world in which we live will catch up with you one day. (Does anyone else feel nostalgia for a good ol', reliable typewriter?)

While you take all the steps you can to maintain control of your own affairs, it is important, as well, to identify and recruit a capable and trustworthy advocate. When it comes to dealing with doctors or resolving problems on an invoice, my daughters are many times more effective than I am. I feel lucky to have two daughters who are ready, willing, and able to drop everything and come running when Charlie or I call.

But here is the secret: Calling for help should be the *exception*, not the rule. If you respect your advocate's busy schedule and separate life, he or she will know that when you call for assistance, it's important.

If you don't have a family member nearby or one up to this task, perhaps you could search out a younger friend—maybe someone in your church—and invite this person to become familiar with your needs, your routines, your medical contacts, even your expectations. Then if you only call when you really need help, chances are that your friend will gladly jump in for you.

It also behooves us to get our affairs in the best order possible so as to make the job of helping us easier for our advocates (as well as for ourselves).

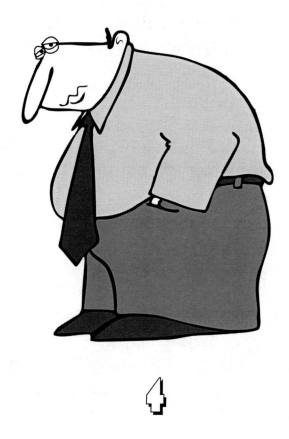

4

MOOD LIFTERS

Challenge is the name of the game at this age, and staying upbeat can become a huge challenge all its own.

The second highest hurdle for us over-the-hill folks may be how to cope with the lowness of spirit (depression) that frequently comes with the territory. Another few lines of poetry come to mind:

Seldom can the heart be lonely
If it seeks one lonelier still,
Self-forgetting, seeking only
Emptier cups with love to fill.
—*Frances Ridley Havergal*

We may be limited in what we are able to do by the situation nature bestows upon us, but there is always something we can offer someone who is left with less. If you still drive, I'll bet you know someone who needs a ride to a doctor's office or the drug store. For a special treat, take a friend to the beauty shop to have her hair done.

Even a quick trip to the grocery store breaks a day's tedium and creates a few minutes for companionable chat. Maybe you could share a casserole you made or a piece of pie, or divide up something someone made for you. These demonstrations of love may be the best medicine of all.

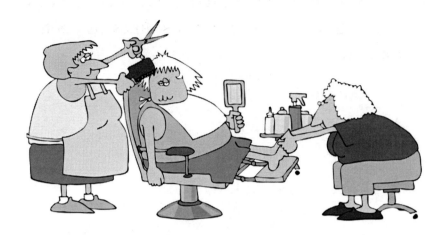

I've routinely corresponded with a lifelong friend for the last several years. Her handwriting is no longer legible, and if not for my computer, I'm sure she would have the same trouble with mine.

But I've come to realize that *reading* my message is not what's most important. Simply seeing the newly arrived envelope may give her a little lift—as it does me—just to know I was thinking about her and vice versa.

Every so often I send her a card with a silly animal picture or a photo of breathtaking scenery. I'll admit that sometimes I even recycle a card if the picture is good enough.

A simple phone call may lift the spirit of someone who has no one with whom to talk or visit. Alexander McIntosh Buchan reminds us, "They also serve who only sit and listen." So the tale you hear is tedious? Count your blessing that your hearing still works!

Giving evidence that someone cares is the point, regardless of the value of actual gifts or services. But I'll let you in on a surprising secret: Remembering to plan and carry out these gestures for others will surely add to your own spirit of well-being every bit as much as it does to theirs.

Before we leave the topic of lifting spirits, I would like to interject a thought about medications for depression. Any decision about medication must be one between you and your doctor(s)—that goes without saying. Nevertheless, some folks in our generation attach a stigma to the mere notion of an antidepressant and resist taking one for this reason alone.

Medications have come a long way during our lifetimes, and many of our peers find that antidepressant medications truly help them

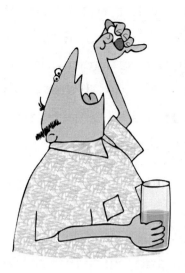

cope better—and more happily—as they come face-to-face with the challenges of age.

In my way of thinking, whatever I can do to stay cheerful, useful, and not a nuisance deserves my un-biased consideration.

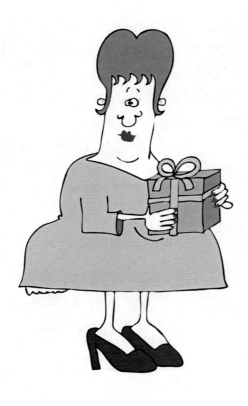

5

PASSING IT ON

Remember learning the following verse from Acts 20:35 in Sunday School?

"It is more blessed to give than to receive."

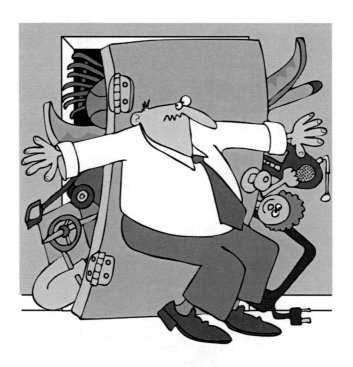

Late in life one of my friends found herself alone in a big, fine home that was chock-full of nice things she had treasured over the years. As her faculties weakened, her first concern shifted from taking care of her accumulation of stuff to taking care of herself.

Her solution was exceptional! She hosted a large family gathering, a party if you will. She issued each guest an appropriate share of play money, and thereafter, she spent the evening auctioning off belongings she would have no need of, or place for, in her chosen care facility, while saving a few extra-special keepsakes.

Sure, there was a small element of sadness to the occasion, but it gave her an opportunity to enjoy the giving, something she would have missed entirely had her belongings been divided up willy-nilly and handed out later by someone who might never have known their value to her. She had great fun passing along special facts or memories with each treasure. These details would have been lost at her passing but added extra value in the hands of the new owner.

While we're on the subject of giving, why not consider going about it a different way? Imagine yourself handing out big and little things of yours to someone dear and enjoying it! For instance, how many more formal dinners do you expect to host? Is there someone among your family or friends who would cherish the fine china collecting dust in your cupboards?

Who might enjoy using your good glassware whether or not it's crystal? Is there a young person in your world with the elbow grease to maintain and the lifestyle to enjoy the sterling silver turning black behind your cabinet doors?

Or try this. You might be surprised how much fun it could be for you if a friend admires something of yours, and you smile, pick it up, and hand it over saying, "I want you to have it!" You'll experience the bonus pleasure of seeing the startled receiver's face.

I have begun placing special family keepsakes with loved ones—my daughters, my grandchildren, my friends. I think there's more pleasure left in them this way than just hanging on to them. If you try it, you will see.

We have noticed a number of items lounging around our household we used to think important but aren't now. If you mentally inventory your belongings, you might find quite a few things you hadn't thought of as givable.

For instance, I am parceling out the seashells from my collection to the kids at our church. Every Sunday, they show up with eager faces to receive one from my pocket. Maybe it will be the stimulus for a lifelong collection of their own. Next, I plan to see if anyone cares about interesting rocks; if so, I'll parcel them out from my rock collection too.

At this point, we will miss neither shells nor rocks, nor various other odds and ends like chopsticks, Japanese fans, small interesting books, toys—all the minutiae and little souvenirs gathered over a lifetime, too good to toss but of little real value. I'm hoping to spare my daughters a big part of the task of sorting and giving away a lifetime of collectables one of these days, and in the process, I get to enjoy the recipients' happy faces.

In this vein, now is a good time to sort and toss. Keep what's important, give what's good, donate what's useful, and toss the rest. Make a list of things you are still using but have promised to someone else when you can no longer use them.

Do you really want to leave your children with half a century or more of trash to sort? Most times, family members will appreciate this help.

A WORD OF CAUTION

Before you get carried away in passing things on, don't forget to bring any heirs, advocates, and estate advisors into the discussion. Provide them with an opportunity for special requests, questions, and input.

It is a reality that our judgment may not always be sound, and there are those who target and prey on our weaknesses. You don't want your treasures to fall victim to any poor oversight on your part or clever cons on others' parts.

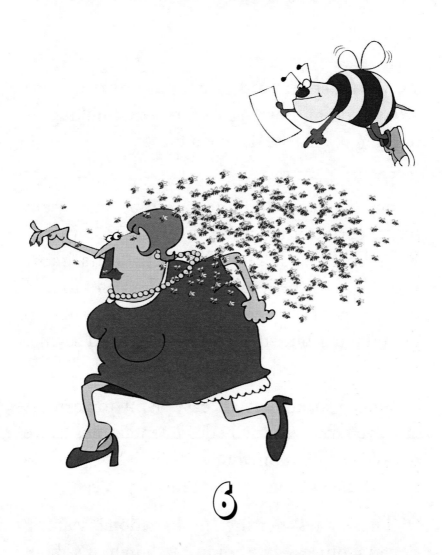

6

Don't Just Sit There, DO Something!

I'm not saying that keeping busy is easy. In fact, staying appropriately busy may be one of the most difficult things we have to do. Even so, we must resist the inclination to just sit around, doing nothing, and mostly thinking of nothing . . . maybe dozing a bit.

If you don't feel well or you don't have anything urgent to do, doing nothing may seem like a perfectly natural or acceptable "activity." But the fact is, just sitting there is habit forming, and the resulting boredom and lack of movement may eventually leave you unable to do anything but sit. Remember the old saying: Move it or lose it!

Sitting around is an easy habit to form at any age but is especially detrimental to us as we get older. Summon your self-discipline, and do something as much of the time as you can.

These days, getting my hair done, visiting doctors' offices, and going to church are about all the going out I do. Remembering and arranging to stay busy the rest of the time is a real challenge. I am thankful for the activities I began arranging a few years ago, and it would have been even better had I started a few years before that. If you wait until you are in your 80s or 90s to begin planning, you may regret it.

Now do I hear you asking, "Do something? Like what?" Reading the previous chapter, *Passing It On*, might have given you a few ideas. But there are lots of other things you can do that are simple and far less ambitious than hosting a giveaway bash.

Take a stab at the puzzles and games found in most newspapers: Sudoku, word search, and crosswords, for example. All these are good to keep our brains from going rusty, and it doesn't matter one whit if we are able to finish them. Pick one, or try your hand at all of them. Any day, it surely beats thumb twiddling.

Remember as a youngster how exciting it was to open a new jigsaw puzzle? Whether tidily laying all the pieces face up, or dumping them in a pile and shuffling through, it all depends on your personal style (and usually summoned a minor disagreement in our family). Fitting in a piece or two or twenty can still fill dabs of time on long days. Some of the newest puzzles are really interesting, many even made in 3-D. While the big, thick pieces may be easy to handle, don't be fooled. These puzzles are tough! You'll definitely get a mental workout. Still, harder isn't necessarily better. Even simple puzzles with large, kind-to-the-eyesight pieces keep fingers and brains active.

How about digging out that old deck of cards and renewing your hand at a game of Solitaire? Truth told, it had been so long since I'd played that my daughter had to give me a refresher course. But now Charlie and I spend many an hour happily engaged in this pastime.

To make it more interesting, we keep an on-going record of our winnings and losings as if we play at a fancy Las Vegas casino. Every hand "costs" $52 and "pays" $5 for each card played at the top. I've played more than 2,670 hands and won a whopping on-paper sum of $12,257 sitting at the card table in my den! Maybe I'll jet off to Paris. Then again, maybe not; I'll take my fun right here at home.

It came as a pleasant surprise to us that Solitaire can be a shared activity, played companionably though not competitively. My husband and I sit side-by-side at the card table, each involved with a separate game, keeping an individual, running score. It's hard not to point out (Charlie calls it refereeing) a move he's overlooking. No doubt it's my help that puts him ahead of me. He's won $37,884 since his last birthday, though I admit the winnings are hard to spend.

From time to time, Charlie brings a friend who's living in a nursing home for a visit, and the three of us sit around the table and play our individual hands—each at his or her own speed and capability. The cards give us a focus for companionable silence as well as a topic of conversation to be easily set aside if better ideas for talk arise. Being together at the same table and making comments to one another enhance the company as well as the game.

Consider setting up a relatively permanent activity center, like a bridge table. Let games and various other activities stay out for easy return later. Place your activity center nearby enough to be handy (but not enough so you'll trip over it). Keep your game supplies boxed and stored at arm's reach. If you have just a wee bit of time, you can play a quick hand or fit a puzzle piece or two into place. If you have a small project underway, this is a good place to work on it, a bit at a time. Any of these activities, even engaged in for just a few minutes, beats just sitting there.

For lots of years I have played matron of the photo albums in our family. By my tally I have made more than thirty books for our daughters, grandchildren, and friends. Admittedly, I may not get the timelines exactly right, but my daughters assure me that having all the old photos tidily displayed in an album—even if they're out of order—vastly improves pictures stored loose in a shoebox. Even in these days of digital photos, I'll bet your loved ones have plenty of the old-fashioned kind eagerly awaiting display.

Working with the photos is a great way to resurrect memories and fond feelings. Since I can no longer write legibly, I use my computer to make labels and interesting little notes to cut-and-paste on the pages. Not only does the activity bring me pleasure, but also it keeps my hands and mind busy. My daughters tell me that my making the albums is the most valuable gift I can give them.

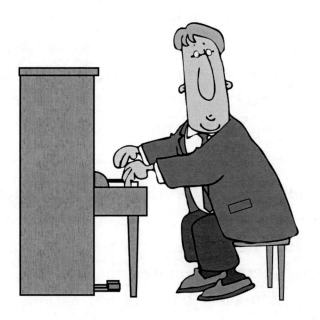

An activity Charlie enjoys fairly regularly is bringing together a few (usually old) folks for a little pickin' and grinnin'. He's always been a man fond of a musical instrument. He fashioned his first guitar out of an orange crate when he was 13 and played in a band when he was in the service. But his love of an instrument eventually took backstage to family raising and career.

For his 87th birthday we gave him an electric guitar. Now he gets together with a few friends—even some young friends from our church seem to enjoy taking a break from their hectic lives—to share a little music. Maybe there's not much music made but certainly plenty of noise and lots of laughter. Did you enjoy playing an instrument once? Why not pick it up again?

It's not too late for a new hobby either. A few years ago, our younger daughter spent some time in a nicely furnished home in England where she enjoyed the use of an unusual wooden salad bowl. It was exceptionally large but tapered down to a very small bowl-like bottom that could serve, with a pestle, in blending a salad dressing. When she returned home, she asked Charlie if he knew anyone who could make one like it.

He did but the woodworker said, "You wouldn't want to pay what it would cost." So, what did he do? He bought an expensive new lathe and made it himself.

Shortly thereafter, a flowering apple tree in the local churchyard gave up the ghost. In preparation for removing it, someone had cut off a fairly large limb and left it on the ground. It tempted Charlie who took it home and made a number of delightfully crafted, beautifully finished nut and candy bowls. He gave these to the church staff so they could remember the little tree that bloomed in the churchyard for so many springs before.

These were inspiration for many more, still active years of woodworking: platters, bowls (with or without creative lids), cheese trays, candlesticks, and lamps that he gives away regularly. He has made several baptismal fonts, and he and a church friend have spent many a fine hour shopping for material, planning, prepping, and finishing, discussing, debating, and arguing (in good spirit). During this time they created a special storage rack for the choir's music and an altar with a nice, permanent stand to hold the open Bible in the small chapel recently added at our church.

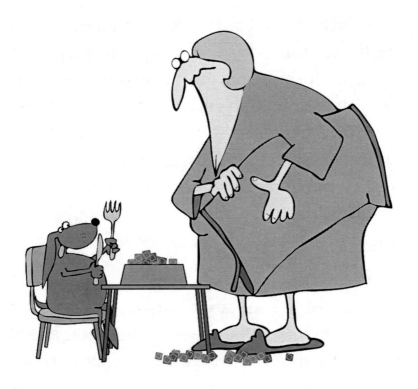

7

TAKE CARE OF
SOMETHING BESIDES
YOURSELF

On our kitchen wall hangs a little wooden
sign reading, "Everyone needs a furry friend."

Charlie and I give that a loud "Amen!" If you are already a pet owner, you understand the value of a dog or cat that knows he or she is yours and seems to worship you. A pet is company, a terrific foil to loneliness. Even a fish can be company. Our granddaughter swears her goldfish, Bobo, greets her every morning by rushing to the side of the bowl and wagging its flipper, and her mother confirms it.

I am reminded of an experience I had with my dad when I was about ten. We were attending an exhibit of army equipment near the city lake when my daddy stumbled across a nest of baby bunnies in danger of being run over by the tanks. Without a second thought, he gathered them up and took them home.

He prepared a tiny bottle for them but found they wouldn't accept it. Although it was nearly midnight by then, Daddy put the bunnies in a box and drove them the ten miles or so back to the spot near the lake. He searched with a flashlight until he located the remains of their nest. He left them there, hoping the mother would return and find them safe.

We never knew their outcome, but Daddy believed, as do I, that caring about animals enhances one's later, slower years. Time spent tending to another creature's needs is worth the effort to both them and us.

A pet gives you something outside of yourself to feel valued by—maybe loved by. It's something important to think about, care about, and tend to. And it definitely gives you something to do!

Only the truly ambitious should bite off what we've bitten off with Winnie and Pooh. Did I hear myself ask again, *What were we thinking?* But seriously, these rowdy little varmints bring a great deal of joy to our days along with quite a few laughs.

There's even more to this pet idea than just the pleasure one brings. Our kitty Widget also served as our household scapegoat. Any faux pas neither of us was eager to claim became Widget's. "Widget must have done it" was to us an acceptable, no-blame excuse for anything that went awry. Then we just let it go—forgot about it and moved on.

If a pet doesn't work for you, you can still . . .

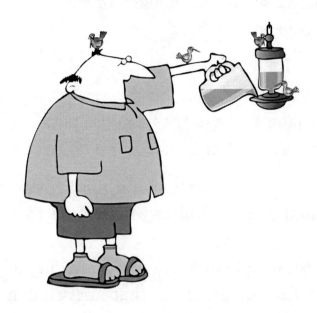

Feed Something. . .

My hometown didn't have a zoo. Instead, people came to our house on Sunday afternoons to see what variety of varmints my dad had amassed during the prior week. They might find a litter of baby gophers in a tub on the porch or a bunny running loose in the house. There were plenty of cats and dogs, but they mostly stayed outside. Many came to know Tat the Rat I raised from a bottle, but the doctor who called to treat me once when I was sick refused to come in the room because he couldn't stand the thought of the pet rat under the covers at my feet.

So I guess you can say animal loving runs in my genes and may be the reason my brother Joey later had a deer as a house pet. (I'll bet you didn't know deer love to jump on the bed!)

You don't have to be a multi-generational animal nut to find it worthwhile to feed the birds, squirrels, stray cats and dogs, and even an occasional possum or raccoon in the neighborhood. I feed anything that arrives at my door hungry. Silly as it sounds, it makes me feel important and needed. Each in its unique way, the little critters provide a strong dose of entertainment as well.

Every day at two o'clock, just after a siesta, I step through the back door to find a driveway filled with dozens of birds, mostly pigeons, and squirrels waiting for me.

I toss out a handful of birdseed and bread bits to the pigeons. More fly in to join the party, and in a heartbeat the drive is blanketed with feasting feathered friends. Some of the "regulars" I have named, such as Bill-N-Coo and several Limpin' Ladies. One squirrel is Brokie Tail, and most of them know what I mean when I call, "Come and get it, squirlie, squirlie!"

I keep a bucket of old pecans on hand for the squirrels. As a special treat, I serve them Ritz crackers which, judging from their response, appear to be squirrel delicacies. The animals are so cute, taking the cracker from my hand with surprisingly human-like hands and spinning it like the turn of a steering wheel, all the while nibbling round the edges until the cracker disappears. A dozen or so visit Oldfield Café every day. I think we look forward to seeing each other.

The half-hour or so spent feeding them gives double purpose with the benefits of the time spent daily out in the bright light.

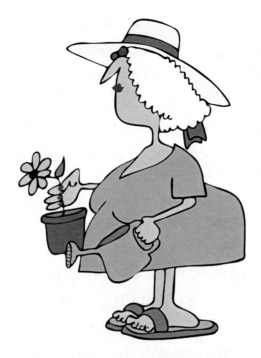

. . . Or Grow Something

If animals aren't your thing, how about a less demanding living thing—a plant? Did you ever catch a sweet potato sprouting in your pantry? I'll bet you cut off the end and threw it away or tossed the whole potato. Had you chosen instead to set it in a bit of soil and water it, you might easily have created a monster. Honest. Sometimes these plants grow so fast you can almost watch them grow. The sprout becomes an attractive indoor vine in no time.

When things might otherwise get pretty dull, I might tack a few shoots to the wall, so they grow this way and that, creating a living tapestry. It might not earn me a spot in *House Beautiful,* but watching the sweet potato vine change day by day brings us joy.

Even tending one small plant by the back door is a manageable task that can make you feel needed!

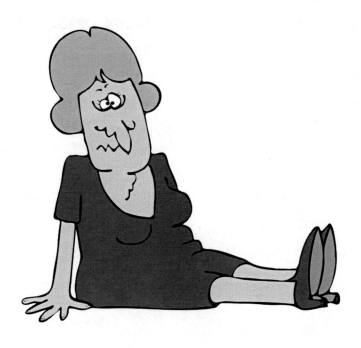

8

SLOW DOWN A BIT

In my early 80s I took a tumble from which I never fully recovered. By now, I've gone down a dozen times, resulting in broken bones, black eyes, a torn rotator cuff, and more. Much discomfort and countless colorful bruises were the outcomes. Experience qualifies me to say falls are not fun, and they are definitely not funny in the way comedy routines might suggest. What makes it worse as we age is that many of us have become exceptionally breakable too.

Slowing down is the most important step in the prevention of falls. The warning to slow down is so important that perhaps it should be tattooed on both wrists! (I wonder what my grandchildren would say if I showed up with a tattoo?) Slowing our pace might let us grab onto a doorframe or at least minimize the damage from the fall if we don't.

Almost as important when we walk is to watch carefully where each of our footfalls will land. Old ladies like me can trip on flowers in the carpet or other stuff not even there.

Try walking with your hand along the wall for that wee touch of added balance. Use handrails; they're there for good purpose.

Oh, and don't try standing on one foot while using the other to snap a cardboard gift wrapping tube to fit it in the trash. I tried that; it

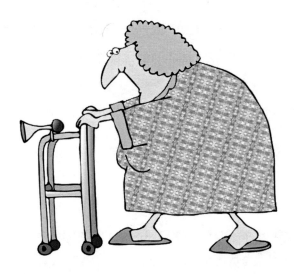

didn't work out so well. The fall resulted in a broken hip that still causes lingering reminders.

A fall is the downfall for many. Few things are more important for us oldsters to avoid. Remember the bit about the old gentleman who had fallen and was being questioned by someone hoping to help. "How did you fall?" The man glumly answered, "Down."

Slow Down, but Don't Stop!

A good friend from childhood, who regularly corresponds with me, frequently mentions her need to "get back to water exercises." She believes the exercise would help her feel more like herself—more like she used to.

Here's the problem with her comment: We can seldom go back at this point. Our time becomes occupied coping with today's problems. The trick is:

DON'T QUIT DOING THE THINGS YOU HOPE TO KEEP DOING!

Charlie still walks two miles most days and plays golf as often as he can corral a partner or two. Most men of his age dropped out of 18-hole contention long ago. But Charlie just keeps on keepin' on. Our daughter and son-in-law include him in golf rounds, and meanwhile, he stays on the lookout for younger and younger men to play with him.

The past four years, he's organized a foursome for our church golf tournament, and his team has won once and placed second twice!

(Charlie insists he's not a sandbagger. Rather the mulligans he buys—with proceeds going to charity—provide a little handicap help!)

Charlie is able to continue doing these and other things because he did them when he was younger and just never quit. During a large part of his working life he rose early every day to walk or jog. By his reckoning, he's logged a lifetime total of 12,000 miles—enough to take him to Istanbul and back! It shows now in so many good ways.

I used to walk with Charlie, but after my first fall and lengthy recovery filled with complications, I didn't restart. Now I wish I could walk with him, but I don't believe I could walk two miles if my life depended on it. Still, I must ask myself if my inability today is because I didn't start again—even a few steps a day—gradually building back up? I honestly don't know, but the result is the same: I can't, or at least, I no longer think I can. My nose may run a good bit these days, but that doesn't get me very far.

Earlier, we talked about the "big if"—if you

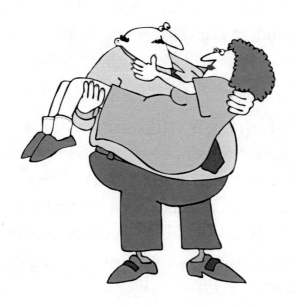

can. Along the way, I realized a very important distinction. *If I can* is different from *if I want to*. I don't want to walk just for exercise when I don't need to go anywhere. *I'm tired.* I don't want to get up and fix dinner. *I'm not hungry.* Believe me, I am a master at excuses of why *I can't* when what I really mean is that *I don't want to*. As the line between *can* and *want* blurs, an I-think-I-can attitude may be all that keeps me going.

If you do try to go back to what you did before, start small and work your way up. Don't expect to pick up where you left off. Don't be hard on yourself or disappointed. Whatever you manage to do is still better than doing nothing at all.

Though many pursuits are behind me now, may I share the benefit of hindsight and suggest to those still able: Don't give up on a valued activity. Especially resist "taking a break" that you tell yourself is temporary. Almost any activity you enjoy will be lost unless you hang in there, keepin' on.

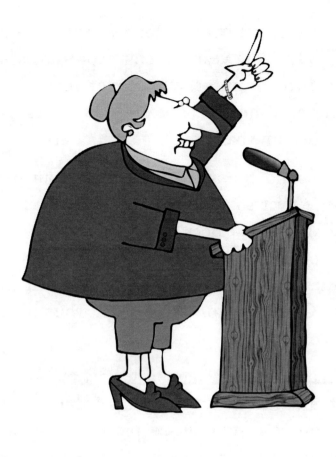

9

FOCUS ON THE BIG STUFF

Because it feels as if we of the older generation are surrounded by nothing but insignifi-
cant doin's, it is important for us to remember

Dr. Carlson's advice: "Don't sweat the small stuff!" Over the years several expressions have come into popularity: "Never mind," "So what?" and more recently, "Who cares?" All carry the same basic message: It doesn't matter.

It's sound counsel. Why elevate your blood pressure over something of little or no importance? Do you or does anyone else really care if your socks don't quite match? If you run two minutes late anywhere but to your own wedding? Or if you forgot to spray your hair, or even comb it?

That said, I do have a hard time keeping quiet about some of the things I think *are* big: 1) the morals and values depicted as normal on television; 2) the flagging support for (real) families; and 3) the greed permeating many institutions. About these issues, I write letters— to the offenders, to the networks, to editors, to stores carrying a particular product, and to my representatives in government.

For years, I've tried to let my voice be heard. It may not change anything in the final analysis, but I haven't sat idle, tacitly approving.

I live in hope that one day enough of us will speak up to be heard. And meanwhile, it gives me something to do!

There are plenty of things we have no ability or power to change. When trouble we can't avoid or fix comes our way, we need to try and put it out of our mind. I'm a worrier of the first order, so I know this advice is much easier said than done. What works for me in this situation is to consciously ask myself two questions:

1) Is this really important?

2) If so, can I do anything about it?

Take it easy; don't be ashamed of pursuing the easy route. Embrace your "who cares" attitude, shrug, and smile. You may find it works wonders for you too.

Or Focus on the Small . . .

Charlie remembers the first time an airplane flew over the little farm where he lived. He and his family stopped their work in the cotton field, looked up, and watched in awe from the moment the plane first appeared overhead until it disappeared on the other side of the sky.

Afterward a sense of eager anticipation grew: when might such a wonder appear again? And when that rare day came, once again everyone would stop what they were doing and stare at the flying craft until it disappeared in the distance.

It never hurts to choose to spend some of our time actively focusing on the joys of the world around us and enjoying the small stuff.

. . . And Dare To Be Odd

I was a Boy Scout. My dad was scoutmaster, and well, at that time it worked better for him if I just joined his troop. Mother helped Daddy, however unofficially, as assistant scoutmaster. In this unorthodox position she taught me a lot about earning merit badges. So when the boys complained it was too hard, mother was quick to point at me and say, "She's doing it!" This, of course, made me very popular with those fellows. (Yeah, right!)

Being a female Boy Scout couldn't have been easy, so it is no small wonder that I was and probably still am a bit odd. No one seemed surprised the day I returned home from school proudly showing off the snake I'd captured with my bare hands. I cried like my heart was

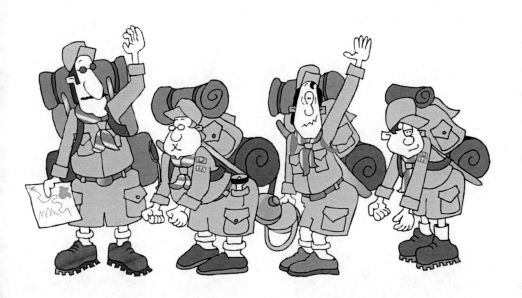

broken when Daddy pried the four-foot treasure from my grip only to discover I had strangled the poor thing on my way home.

Remember and cherish the stories in your own family, the ones that set yours apart from all the others. And share them. You may be surprised how many recurring themes you find when you give yourself permission to embrace your personal history, oddities and all.

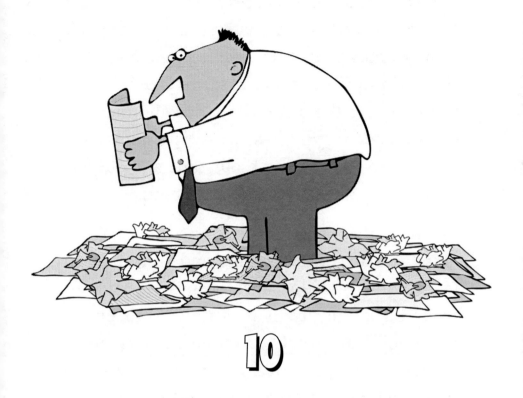

10

REORGANIZE

And the sooner the better. There will be plenty of large, overall matters you'll contend with as you sprint toward your 80s and 90s, but there are also quite a few *little* things you can do now—wherever you are on the timeline—to make a big difference down the road.

While the clock keeps ticking, the actual amount of time we have in a day doesn't change. However, when we become less efficient in using our time, it seems like we have less of it. At the same time, our allotment of energy undoubtedly lessens, so it is important to find ways to save both our time and our energy. Reorganizing can help with both.

Most of us grew up hearing the familiar quip, "A place for everything and everything in its place." It couldn't have been more relevant to us back then than it is now. Your entire household can benefit from an organizational makeover in anticipation of your changing needs before getting around and saving steps become problems. Being prepared can make all the difference in your quality of life.

A Home for Everything

Oftentimes, the "home" for things evolved. An empty place was filled, and we became used to it. The location may work now only because it is familiar and not because it is convenient.

Here's an example of what I mean. One day it occurred to me to wonder why I kept my tweezers in my bedroom dressing table when I almost always used them in the kitchen to organize my 21 pills a day. And why did my hand lotion live in the bathroom? Every time I needed it (often and usually while sitting on the sofa watching television), I had to get up and head down the hall.

Nowadays when the day winds to a close, I usually feel pretty spent and anxious to rest without the ups and downs. So here is my solution: Find a home for things you use frequently within easy reach of the place where you use them. This simple strategy makes a huge difference as the time/energy imbalance grows.

In consideration of a reorganization plan, I have stashed a small plastic box under the edge of the couch where I usually sit. It's hidden from sight so it doesn't mess up the house while still being handy. In it are things like hand lotion, eye drops, cough drops, nail clippers, dental floss—everything I often find myself needing to hop up and retrieve from somewhere else. That little box saves me scores of unnecessary steps. Plus there is an added benefit: I don't have to remember where these things are kept. They'll be right *where* I need them *when* I need them.

Here's another idea: It didn't take many cold nights after a good, hot bath, wandering around a chilly bedroom gathering up my nightclothes to realize I needed a better plan for that too. Charlie added one shelf in a bathroom cabinet, and now everything that goes on and off in the bathroom, including my nightclothes, lives there. Why keep them in the cold bedroom when I need them after a warm bath in the still warm bathroom? Think about it. It works great for me.

Across the span of our six decades of shared household, Charlie and I have amassed eight pairs of scissors that mostly collected themselves in the kitchen drawer where scissors were supposed to live.

On first blush you might ask, "Who in heaven's name needs eight pairs of scissors?" Well, I do.

Have you ever thought about how many ways scissors are used? After some consideration I repositioned most of them, although one pair stayed in the kitchen drawer near our calendar and telephone. One now lives in the computer desk in a back bedroom, another was moved to the prescription/medication box, and others found a myriad of other handy homes. You might consider investing in another pair or two. Scissors cost little compared to the saved steps, not to mention the reduced frustration of searching for a good pair.

And who needs lots of little trash baskets lined with plastic grocery bags? I do. I keep five or six strategically placed around the house with a supply of bags in the bottom as refills. Easily emptied and refilled by slipping out one bag and replacing with another, they make everyday living much tidier.

Are you looking for something to do? Consider carving out some time to find more convenient homes for the things you use often. If you wait too long to start, you may no longer have the energy or ingenuity to do it.

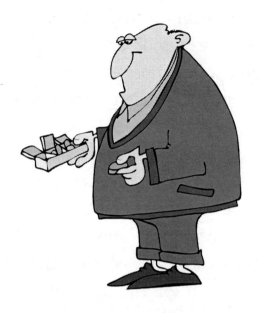

Reorganize Yourself

It is many times worth the effort to reorganize, but to get started we need discipline. The word discipline may call to mind school children in trouble or spankings from a time before they became taboo, but discipline is something we oldsters need too—self-discipline.

Seldom will we find ourselves wanting to do the things that may be best for us. We want what we want whether it's good for us or not. We tend to feel as if we deserve it so a strong dose of self-discipline is usually required. We may choose just to sit around most of the time, but doing something—anything—is better for us than doing nothing. Whatever comes along, we need to be mature enough to trust our thinking cap instead of our wishbone.

It's important at our age that we hold ourselves accountable because no one else is likely to do it. (We are holding our own, remember?) And even if they did, we would probably resent them for doing so.

Keep Your Eye Out for Work-Arounds

Much as I hate to admit it, there is probably something to the idea that we become set in our ways as we age. Habits and routines can be helpful, but remaining open-minded and flexible can definitely bear fruit too.

Start watching for alternative ways to go about doing something. If you are already noticing that certain things are becoming more difficult, don't ignore these early warning signs. Rather, embrace them as a chance to change your habits now, while you still can.

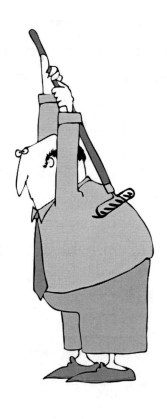

Is handwriting becoming more challenging? Take a deep breath, screw up your courage, and give word processing a go before it's too late.

I have learned to make the type big and easy on my eyes (what a gift!) and even highlight some of it in color. My inexpensive keyboard with extra large letters makes it even easier. If you learn how to use these gadgets now, you will be able to carry these skills well beyond the time you would have lost the dexterity to write.

Have you tried an electronic reader yet, like an iPad or a Kindle? Me neither. But my daughters are insisting I try it, hoping I can again enjoy reading for pleasure given the ability to enlarge the type as needed.

For folks whose vision is seriously impaired, there are lots of books on tape. Learn to read with your ears while you still have the ability to grasp the technology involved.

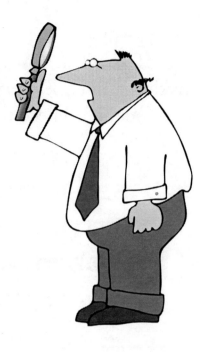

Are you losing your sense of taste? Well, why not look at your situation as an opportunity to help maintain (or regain) a more slender figure.

My mother always said, "There is more than one way to skin a cat." This is true in spades for us oldsters, if we are willing to give new technologies a try. But we can't wait too long! All it takes is finding someone who will help us to master the new possibilities of our day and then giving them a try in our everyday lives. (Maybe I will have my daughter help me test out that new iPad!)

Other Ways To Organize

You will give yourself a great gift for the future if you learn now to be diligent about making a note of everything you will (or suspect you might) need to remember.

BE A JOTTER-DOWNER, A LABELER, AND A SAFEKEEPER OF BOTH THE JOTS AND THE LABELS.

If your memory is dependable today, it may be hard to realize it may let you down tomorrow. Having a written reminder gives you a backup plan and may even allow you to keep it to yourself that your own built-in reminder system isn't working as well as it once did.

If you cement the habit of jotting something down before you start forgetting, you can feel assured important stuff will not be forgotten. By keeping these notes in the same, handy place all the time, you won't forget where the list is. To accomplish this goal, you'll want to have a writing pad at your fingertips.

Accepting the fact that you will forget (Don't we all at any age?) gives you permission not to feel silly labeling familiar things and making lists before you actually need to do so. If you're going to store a box on a high shelf, doesn't it make more sense to label it with large letters before putting it up there? In the future you'll be able to tell what's inside without lifting it down time and again, perhaps risking life or limb by climbing on a chair or shaky footstool.

Before consigning a container of leftovers to the freezer, it's easy as pie to make a wee label and attach it to the lid with a dab of rubber cement. Rather than finding a mysterious dish of questionable lineage, you'll know you have "Chicken Tortilla 2/23" or "Pork Chops & Rice 8/16." Time to eat or time to toss? There will be no doubt what to do.

One of my daughters has commented how much she appreciates a gift from the mother-in-law she never had the privilege of knowing.

Inside each of her mother-in-law's jewelry boxes was pressed a handwritten note telling a bit about the piece's history. The jewelry was modest but the contents grew more precious for the moments of life shared in those notes.

Hoard Good, Sturdy Boxes

It's never too early to start, and if the sight of the boxes offends you, make it part of your "do something" regimen to cover them with scraps of pre-pasted wallpaper or gift wrap, sticky-backed shelf paper, or even spray paint. On the other hand, clear plastic boxes are a boon because they are inexpensive, long-lasting, and you can view the contents easily.

Lightweight boxes are easily moved from place-to-place and manage small items so that they are out of sight but handy. They are definitely key tools in organization. Little woven baskets work well too, holding mail needing to be answered, greeting cards, or photos.

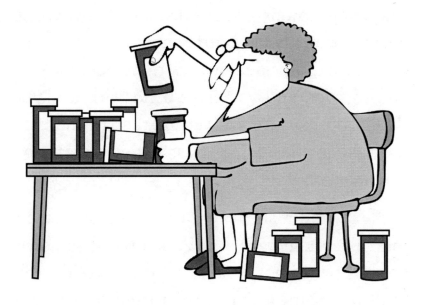

11

TAKE CONTROL OF MEDICATIONS

Managing medicines is no easy task, and mistakes can be problematic if not dangerous. If you are like most of us old folks, you take many pills.

Here is a great tip I learned from a therapist who came to our house once. She showed me that most medicine bottles now have lids that work as well upside down as right side up. Flip the lid over, and you have a lid with a blank slate. You can use a black marker to indicate the medicine inside, or you can glue an easy-to-read label on it.

Next, find a small box with a lid and stand the pill containers inside. When you look down on the opened box, you'll find it easy to identify each medication. No need to pull out bottle after bottle to read small labels. This organization makes transferring meds to a weekly/daily pill dispenser much easier. Store the closed box holding all your medicines in a handy but out-of-sight spot near where you refill your dispensers until it's time to do so.

Prepare a typed list of the medications you take and keep this list up to date. Note when, why, how much, and a description of each, and keep a copy in your box. When you refill your weekly dispensers, it is much easier—and more reliable—to work from this reference than to draw from memory while trying to read each label. Your easy-to-follow medication list will also be of great help to others if a time comes (and it probably will) when you need help with your medications.

Incidentally, if you fill two seven-day dispensers at once, you virtually cut the work in half. This will help you keep tabs on your supply, and you'll reduce the risk of running out of an important medication at an inopportune moment such as when you have no way of getting to the pharmacy.

Medical Reference List

You can greatly simplify visits to the doctor and/or the emergency room if you also keep a copy of your current list of medications in your purse or wallet.

On the reverse side of the medication sheet, I list my major medical conditions and important medical history. I also include the names of all my doctors and specialists with their office phone numbers. When I check in at the doctor's office or the hospital and give them the list to copy, they have most everything they need. And I don't have to remember or write down anything at all!

You'll be especially glad you have this handy document when an ailment prompts your visit to the doctor, and you are not feeling up to doing paperwork. If you should be unconscious, a handy, current medical reference list could literally become a lifesaver. Emergency personnel, your family, and your advocate need to have ready access to this vital information so they can move things quickly toward your treatment and recovery.

Build Your Own Necessity Bag

I don't know what a male equivalent might be, but for my fellow ladies I suggest assembling a small, zippered necessity bag that can fit inside your purse and go anywhere with you. Since I spend most of the day in the den I keep it there, but I carry the bag with me to the bedroom when I retire for the night. In this way

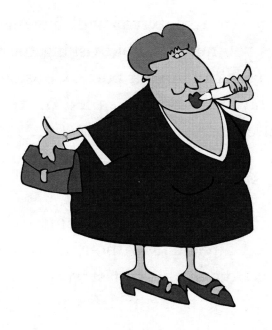

my small needs are always met easily. My bag contains things like a hearing-aid holder, a small battery tester and batteries, a small dental plate holder, my glasses and lens cleaner, one day's medications plus pain pills, lip ointment, eye drops, dry-mouth cough drops, dental floss, tiny paper tablet, pen, and pencil, the afore-mentioned medical reference list—every little thing you might need often, throughout the day or night at home or especially elsewhere.

If you've made a trip to the emergency room, you know they instruct you to leave your purse behind. A necessity bag is the perfect compromise. In a snap, you will have all the little things you need without risking the valuables you may carry in your purse. Consider too that one day you may be called on to help someone else when you least expect it. You'll be prepared to take care of yourself without burdening or delaying the situation.

I would have multiple problems if I ever found myself anywhere without my necessity bag—just as I did at church last week. I had accidentally left it at home—what a mess I found myself in!

If you are a youngster still in your 60s or 70s still managing your routine tasks with ease, you may find it hard to see the point in some of these suggestions. But from the shoes I fill, I know by experience that helpful habits adopted before you need them will pay off in multiples in helping you with maintenance and independence down the road.

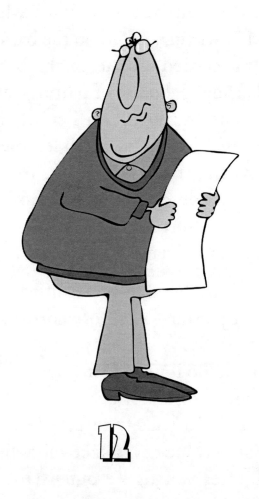

12

DO IT NOW!

Thomas Jefferson is credited with the familiar phrase: "Never put off till tomorrow what can be done today." Most everyone has a to do list of one sort or another, whether for-malized in writing, jotted on the back of an en-velope, or carried around in the back of your head. For me, the habit of putting pen to paper has become invaluable in lieu of short-term memory that has pretty much left me. Plus, the act of writing things down makes my to dos real. I've made a commitment of sorts. If I make a real effort to follow my list, it provides the focus for my day.

As writing became more difficult for me, I devised a personal form of shorthand. For ex-ample, UP NOW means pick up, put up, and tidy up, and do it now. Don't put it off (don't let it pile up) until tomorrow if it's on today's list. Moreover it isn't likely to take less time or be easier later. It may even take more time and be harder, after you figure out what it was that needed doing in the first place.

Putting off putting away means you and those who share your household live in clutter that increases your risk of falling. And worse, you'll probably often find yourself looking for something because chances are good you'll have forgotten where you left whatever it is you're looking for.

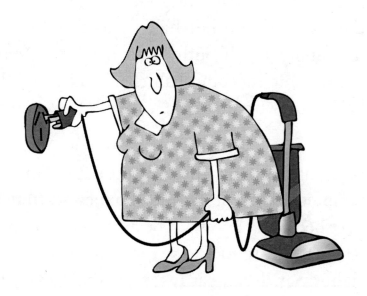

It's a good idea to put items away when you are finished with them. By the end of the day, you may be surprised how much difference this will make in the tidiness of your living area and the control you feel over your surroundings.

Make the most of your while-you're-at-its. Let's say you're headed for the bedroom from the den. Glance around and see if there is anything located where you are that needs to be transported to where you are going—while you're at it. We've found that it makes life so much more simple.

Knowing these are good ideas is only half the story. The other half is planning and reminding yourself until "do it now" and "while-you're-at-it" become habits. If you form these habits, over time you can save a lot of energy.

Say I just finished several hours of work bringing a photo album up to date. Am I ever tempted to just leave the supplies scattered all over because I know I'll be at it again, sooner or later? If I'm tired and really don't want to do it right away, I can easily ignore the mess. But if the supplies have been organized in a sturdy open-top box or two (mounting corners, scissors, paper clips, pens and pencils, rubber cement, etc.), I can slide it all out of sight in seconds. Voila. Tidy. Then I can sit down and feel more at peace.

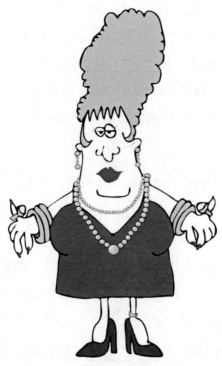

You look mahvelous!

RANDOM THINK-ABOUTS

Beware of Ugly!

A greeting card from my daughter on my 77th birthday read, "OLD AGE ain't so bad.

It's UGLY you have to watch out for." The quip was good for a laugh at the time, but these days I cringe each time I pass a mirror. It's a good thing most folks around us are glad to cut us some slack in the beauty arena; in all likelihood, we are our own worst critics.

While others may not seem to care, our appearance does affect the image they have of us as well as the image we have of ourselves. Cleanliness and tidiness are ideas worth giving some attention. It takes little time or effort to apply a bit of powder, add a touch of lipstick, or tweeze off a few whiskers sprouting where you don't really want them. Showering and wearing clean clothes take a little more effort, but you might be surprised how much better the effort makes you feel. Give it your best shot!

The author of the following little saying is unknown: "Wrinkled was not one of the things I wanted to be when I grew up." There's little I can do about that particular gravitational issue, but there's one thing we can all do to work against it. Remember your mother giving this advice? The prettiest thing to wear is a smile!

Most pictures of Jesus show Him with a serious, sometimes somber expression. I prefer the image of Jesus we have on the wall of our kitchen—Jesus with a great, big, tooth-baring grin. Does it seem likely children would have been drawn to Him, as reported in the Bible, if He didn't laugh or smile fairly often?

If we feel others are pulling away from us perhaps if we smile more often we may find them drawing closer once again.

Make Use of Your Imagination

When we think "ugly" we usually think in physical terms. But other, less-than-attractive issues sometimes go with old age too.

For pity's sake, don't assume that you or your living quarters smell nice. Chances are that somewhere along the way your "smeller" will not be up to par, and you will have nothing to remind you to take care of common odors.

A bath and good housecleaning are important, but beyond these, it's good to assume there are some offensive smells. Use a little cologne or aftershave to mask them. But because your nose is not working well, don't assume you need extra. We certainly don't want friends to smell us before they see us coming!

You can also install one of those automatic room fresheners, which are nice additions even if not exactly necessary. Your friends and family will appreciate them even if you can't.

It's Not Too Late To Have Fun!

Bear with me for a poignant recollection that, believe it or not, really does suit the heading.

Mother was . . . well, different. When I was about six years old, my father took her to Mayo Clinic where she was asked an odd question: "How long do you want to live?"

"Until my daughter is grown, I guess."

"At what age would that be?" she was asked.

"Eighteen, I guess."

The doctor replied, "Then you will need to spend 18 hours a day in bed."

Thus she had little time for friendly gatherings, personal friends, shopping, or other ordinary pursuits mothers and daughters or mothers and their friends might share.

Ours were times of her dreams, and in her limited allotment, she was determined to make a lady out of me—a lady of the big-city, high-society, debutant-style. A lady, she admonished, was one who always puts her toes down first with each step. Try it! You may find yourself feeling less than ladylike, as I did then. (But be careful lest you fall!)

She told me I was named after a relative, Princess Beatrice of England. Whether this piece of lore was a figment of her active imagination or based on fact, I couldn't say. But either way, she certainly wanted the role for me.

She had engraved calling cards made and gave them to me along with detailed instructions of how to leave them on the silver tray when the butler would meet me at the door when I went calling. I never was able to try them out because, to my knowledge, no one in our relatively small town had a butler or even knew what one was.

One day, when I was 18 and mother was 44, she sat up on the side of her bed, leaned into the open window beside it, and called out to me as I headed down the sidewalk, "Have a good time!" These were her last words to me, not that she or I knew it at the time.

I have thought about these words often, and as parting words go, these were good: a simple reminder to enjoy the gift of life.

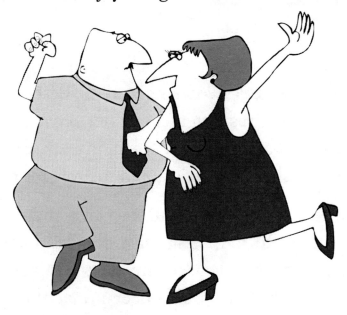

Every day I try to remind myself of mother's reminder to enjoy life. The advice was good. Remember to have a good time and make this your goal even when doing something that isn't fun for you to do!

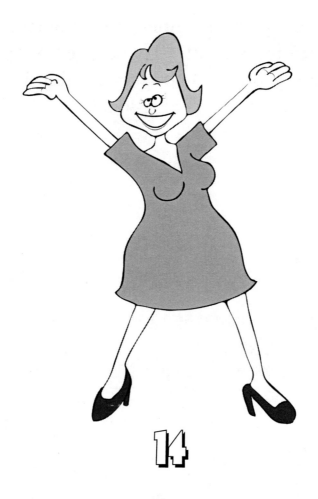

14

THINKING CHEERY!

There is little I need and even less I want in material goods these days. Good times may not be as uproarious as they once were, but we can still find ways to find simple enjoyment.

Knowing my lack of material wants, my younger daughter scratched her head at Christmas-time. Inspiration struck, and who would have thought I could have so much fun with any gift at this point?

I opened the package to find a child's toy. Tickle Me Elmo it was called. We took the fuzzy, red figure from the box and turned it on. Before we knew it, we were all laughing along with Elmo until we cried. Now that was a gift I needed.

Since then, I've had a good time with Elmo, showing him off to any number of visitors with similar results. Now I'm passing him along to a friend who I hope will share the good time with a whole new crop of unsuspecting chucklers in the care home where she is living.

Ponder this little poem:

Laugh and the world laughs with you;
Weep and you weep alone.
For this sad old earth must borrow its mirth,
But has trouble enough of its own.
   —*Ella Wheeler Wilcox*

Consider carrying a joke or a little quip in your pocket, ready at a moment's notice to greet a friend or lighten a mood. A silly little smile-maker gives others—and you—a reason to smile. You might be surprised how eagerly others respond to a light moment. A touch of humor can come in handy as an icebreaker too.

There are many entertaining little books filled with good material. I try to keep several on hand so if someone isn't feeling well or is depressed, I have a ready mood lifter to leave with them. (And they're good for expanding my own repertoire as well!)

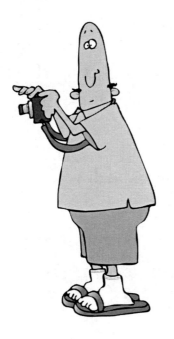

Fred took some vacation photos with a disposable camera but tossed it out before developing the film!

Here are several of my favorite pocket quips. Maybe they're a tad corny, but rarely do I offer one of these that isn't met with a chuckle:

A doctor greeted his patient asking how she was doing.

"Oh, just terrible," she moaned. "I hurt all over." Punching herself vigorously with her forefinger she continued, "This hurts (head), this hurts (throat), this hurts (chest) . . ."

"I know," the doctor replied, nodding wisely.

The patient in surprise answered, "You know? How can you know?"

"I see," said the doctor, "you have a broken finger."

What do you call a male deer that is crazy about female deer?

A doe-nut.

My daughter was recently travelling in South Dakota where real buffalo roamed, and she came back asking: "What did Papa Buffalo say to his boy when he left home?"

"Bye-son."

Two lady friends were motoring down the street, and they ran a red light. The passenger cringed but didn't say anything. Before long, they ran another red light. This time the passenger felt she had to speak up.

Gently she asked her friend, "Did you see that red light?"

"I sure did," replied the driver with some indignation.

"Well then," the passenger continued, "why didn't you stop?"

Her friend paused. "Oh, am I driving?"

Speaking of Driving . . .

Choosing to stop driving is a choice we can make, a voluntary response to change. After a long illness, I realized I could not respond as quickly as I needed to the demands of traffic—so many cars, so much speed. I didn't want to give up my independence, but I equally didn't want to put others at risk because of me. I made the hard decision to stop driving.

We do everyone a favor, ourselves included, if we are honest in evaluating our capacities for handling potentially dangerous situations. This thought process applies also to our living situation—the choice of living alone versus moving where we have some extra assistance or even just company—and keeping ourselves safe.

You will be happier with the decisions if *you* make them rather than if someone at some time is required to force them on you.

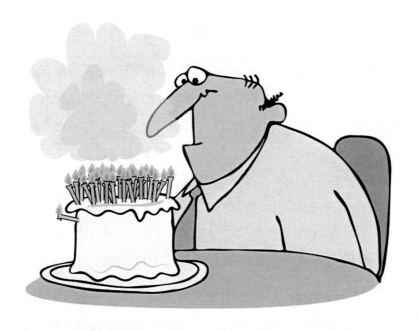

COUNT ON CHANGE

Remember when the price of a hamburger skyrocketed to 15 cents and a time when most of the young women graduating high school were of the sweet-16-and-never-been-kissed variety?

Yep, the times they are a-changin'—and faster than ever before! But perhaps even more important than a changing world to those of us facing our ninth or tenth decade is the change in us. When real old age caught up with Charlie and me, we were surprised how quickly life became different. In fact, about the only constant in my life these days is change.

Like it or not, unexpected changes await us. While we may have no control over them, we can choose how we react. What I know is that I don't know what's coming next, so how do I make the best of it?

We can make faces. We can grin and bear it. We can go with the flow. If I prepare myself for uncertainty, it somehow seems easier to swallow when it shows up on my plate.

Remaining flexible is key. If you expect to make changes, maybe it will be easier to adjust to different circumstances or even find a way to take advantage of them.

Making It Easy

It's worth your time to seek out and learn better (or at least easier) ways to do things you may have done the hard way before. For example, did you know there is a better way for an old lady to get in a car than the usual head-first?

Here's how: Open the car door and put inside your purse or anything you're carrying. Move near the car so your closest leg touches the doorframe. While holding on to the car door, turn your back to the car and shuffle backwards until the calves of your legs are against the door frame. Holding on, sit down sideways in the seat. Pull in your feet and rotate frontward. This way is not only safer, it's also more ladylike. (It works for older gents too.)

Learn to shop by mail through catalogs or on the internet for everything reasonable. When getting around becomes a problem, knowing how to have things you need or want arrive at your front door can definitely make life easier.

Or how about putting your clothes on sitting down? When you get used to it, it's easy. It saves energy, and best of all, you'll be less likely to fall.

Select clothes with pockets. You may even want to add to your wardrobe one or more pocketed, long vests. Pockets are handy at any age but especially when every step seems one too many. Something I use often, like tissues, cough drops, or lip gloss, is many times easier to find in my pocket. It saves countless steps and lots of frustration in hunting when I can't remember where I left it.

Live in the Light

"Brighten the corner where you are" is a multi-pronged suggestion, being good advice both literally and figuratively.

Open your drapes first thing every morning. Even if you don't crave a shot of morning light, your body does. After dark or on a dreary day, remember to turn on more lights.

Living where it is brighter makes it easier for us to see. For some people poor lighting— perhaps more than their worsening eyesight— is leaving them in the dark. It's good to go outdoors and sit on our porches, watching the goings-on for at least 30 minutes. If you have bought into the idea of feeding critters, you can doubly benefit from time outside, not necessarily in the sunlight but at least in the bright daylight.

Paying attention to light and dark also helps us maintain our body clocks. It's no secret that maintaining a reasonably normal day/night schedule contributes to our overall well-being.

Bright colors help too. Nowhere does it say that because we are old we must wear and surround ourselves with drabness. And here's the best part: more light and color may push back the gloominess that tries harder and harder to invade our homes as we grow older. Up your light and color levels, and you may find your spirits lifted too.

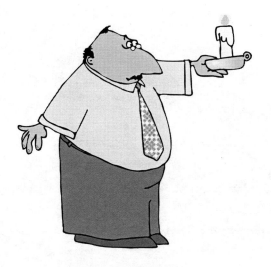

God's Light

I think there may be more than meets the eye to this idea of living in the light, and that's changing to walk even closer in God's light. When our memory goes, as it does in varying degrees for all us oldsters, we may not talk much about our beliefs, but we may find ourselves putting them on a little more tightly around us during the end-time thinking, when we may need them most.

I don't dwell on the next chapter of my life, though at my age it is impossible to ignore it altogether. But I rest peacefully knowing my heavenly Father will leave the light on for me!

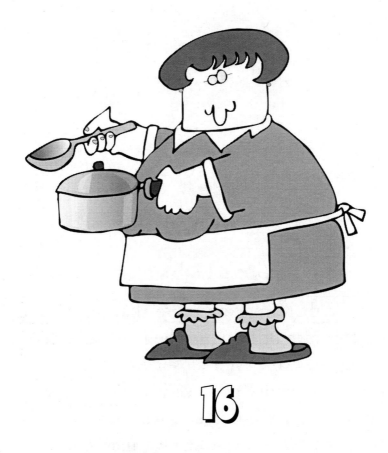

16

A WORD TO THE COOK

It wasn't my intention to write a cookbook, but since eating is a need we share, no matter our age, I dare to add a few bits worth of this and that related to food preparation and how we can simplify the process. We should always try and remember that neglecting healthy eating is sure to lead us into trouble.

If you still prepare your own meals, while you are making one, cook double the amount or more and freeze the extra. (Even better, before you freeze it, divide into meal-sized servings. And don't forget to label and date!)

You can plan, shop for, prepare, and clean up after multiple casseroles, soups, salads, whatever with little more effort than required to fix enough for a single meal. Think how nice it will be to have a warm-and-eat dish at a time when you don't feel up to cooking, don't have enough time to do so, or have company drop in. If I plan and start early, I can find the energy to prepare some of my favorites.

Break down recipes that take a good bit more work—more effort than I am likely to want to put into dinner late in the day. What can you prepare in advance? What can you keep on hand? Tackling a recipe in multiples allows us to keep variety in our meals and preparation under control. Even better, it keeps our all-time favorites in reach.

When preparing a recipe calling for cooked chicken, for instance, I've learned to stew, bone, and skin three or four birds at once. I then divide it six, eight, or even ten ways, and freeze for use in favorite recipes later. Strain and freeze the broth in an extra ice cube tray. (If you don't still have one, they can be bought at a local dollar store.) Once frozen, broth cubes can be put in a freezer bag, and you can have small portions of homemade chicken broth as easily as popping out a cube.

You won't know how well these ideas will work for you until you try them. For me, the convenience and tastiness are well worth the bit of extra effort.

Even though we enjoy variety, we also like easy. Consider narrowing your choices to simple meals of the same dish on the same day each week. This works really well for us. We have bacon, eggs, toast or biscuit, and sugar-free preserves (our favorites) for supper every Monday night. We go to the kitchen together, knowing exactly what we are each going to do, and 15 minutes later supper is on the table, and the cleanup is minimal since we clean up as we go as much as possible. If you tackle meal preparation this way, it becomes more of a game than a chore.

Wednesday is our pizza day. Starting with ready-made frozen pizza, we add the extra toppings we like best. Our "homemade" pizza is on the table 15 minutes later.

After church on Sundays we pick up a favorite ready-made dinner on the way home (usually Chinese). It's enough for us and a live-alone friend to share.

Our "country dinner"—beans, cornbread (from a mix), maybe pork chops or sausage, and cabbage—takes a little longer but the country boy among us thinks it's worth every second of the extra time and effort.

You probably have your own favorites, dishes you like well enough to eat every week. So put on your thinking cap and do your own thing, but plan it ahead for multiple servings.

Of course it's wise to be flexible if something better comes along, but at the same time it is reassuring to know that the regular choice is there, if nothing better presents itself.

While we are talking recipes, I bet you won't mind if I sneak in a few. Back when I was learning to cook, I had never heard of Vegetable Marinade. It's one of our favorite recipes now and easily adjustable to fit dietary limitations or preferences. It's a *QEG.*

QEG

QEG stands for quick, easy, and good. It's my code for preferred recipes. May I suggest you evaluate your own recipes and mark those that qualify so they'll be easy to find.

Going through your recipes again after perhaps many years, you are sure to discover a few old favorites you will be eager to try again.

SUBSTITUTIONS

Substitutions become the order of the day as we adjust to special dietary needs. When you must, use good judgment. Don't be like the lady who was serving a fancy dinner and proudly told her guests the Lobster Bisque recipe had been shared by another guest. This guest was confused and embarrassed because the dish bore no resemblance to hers, and she found it to be less than praiseworthy. So she gently questioned the hostess.

The hostess replied with enthusiasm, "I always tell my guests it's your recipe, but I did have to make a few changes. I couldn't find any lobster so I substituted canned tuna. I needed to cut the calories, so I used chicken soup instead of sour cream. I didn't have any wine so I used a little grape juice. Isn't it yummy?"

VEGETABLE MARINADE

(Serves 12 maybe . . . depending upon what you decide to put in it.)

1 can green beans, French cut, drained

1 can white, shoe-peg corn, drained

1 can Le Sueur peas, drained

1 jar chopped pimiento with juice

½ c. sugar

¾ c. wine vinegar

1 tsp. seasoned salt

1/3 c. salad oil

Mix vegetables in large, sealable container. Heat together sugar, vinegar, salt, and oil. Pour over veggies and mix well. Refrigerate several hours. Serve cold. It's ready at a moment's notice to round out a meal and keeps for 2-3 weeks.

Variations: add mushrooms, water chestnuts, carrots (raw or cooked, grated or chopped), and/or any other vegetables you especially like.

CHICKEN & DUMPLINGS

(Serves 8)

I wanted to include this recipe, which won't be easy since I don't have a recipe! Mostly I make it by-guess-and-by-golly, with a really helpful tip from my brother Joe (1914-1977).

1 chicken, stewed until tender w/celery, onion, salt, pepper (skinned, boned and chopped); reserve broth

1 can of buttermilk biscuits

1 c. milk

Early on the day of serving, open biscuits, and on floured board, roll out each biscuit separately to about 1/8" thickness. Allow them to dry (several hours at least); then cut each one into 4-5 thin pieces. Strain broth and bring to a boil. Add milk. Drop dumplings, 1 slice at a time, into broth. When dumplings are done (taste test), add chicken bits. Thicken broth with cornstarch mixed with a little milk, if desired. Salt and pepper to taste.

TOMATO ASPIC SALAD

(Serves 6)

In case you, like us, love tomatoes but can't eat them because of the seeds . . .

1 pkg. lemon Jell-O (sugar-free if desired)

2 c. tomato juice	½ sm. onion, shredded
1 bay leaf	½ tsp. salt
dash black pepper	2 tbsp. cider vinegar
1 c. celery, chopped	mayonnaise

Heat tomato juice, onion, bay leaf, salt, and pepper to boiling. Strain. Dissolve Jell-O in tomato broth. Stir in vinegar and celery. Chill until set. Just before serving, cut into squares and dab top with a bit of mayonnaise.

Variations: add other vegetables of your choice such as carrots, bell peppers, or water chestnuts.

CRANBERRY CHICKEN

(Serves 8)

8 chicken breast halves (or 22-24 tenders)

garlic powder

8 oz. bottle Russian salad dressing

1 pkg. of dry onion soup mix

16 oz. can whole berry cranberry sauce

Spray 2 qt. baking dish with non-stick spray. Arrange chicken in baking dish and sprinkle with garlic powder. Mix Russian dressing, soup mix, and cranberry sauce. Pour over chicken and marinade overnight (easy for company). Cover with foil and cook 30 min. at 325°. Remove foil and bake another 30 min. Baste if needed (mine seldom does). Let stand in oven 15 min. with oven turned off and door open.

MOCK ORIENTAL CHICKEN

(Serves 4)

2 pks. Ramen Noodle Soup mix

2 c. boiling water

8 oz. cooked chicken (canned is fine)

½ tsp. ginger powder

1 c. broccoli flowerets

1 c. carrots, grated

2 tbsp. sesame seeds toasted in butter
or margarine (optional)

Break up noodles in boiling water. Add one flavor seasoning packet. Cook uncovered for 3 min. Meanwhile, sauté chicken and ginger with second seasoning packet contents. Add vegetables. Combine noodles, chicken mixture, and vegetables, and cook an additional 2 mins. Top with sesame seeds before serving.

JACK STRAWS CASSEROLE

(Serves 6)

1 lb. ground beef, partially browned

1 c. celery, chopped

1 c. onion, chopped

½ tsp. seasoned salt

1 pkg. frozen chopped broccoli

1 can cream of mushroom soup

½ c. milk

1 can shoestring potatoes

Add vegetables and salt to partially browned ground beef and continue cooking until soft. Thin soup with milk. Layer 1/3 meat mixture in bottom of casserole. Add layer of 1/3 broccoli, and then a layer of 1/3 mushroom soup mix. Repeat (three layers). Top with shoestring potatoes and bake uncovered at 350° for 30 min.

OUTSIDE-IN CUPCAKES

(Makes 24 – 30)

8 oz. pkg. cream cheese

1/3 c. sugar

1 egg

¼ tsp. salt

1 tsp. vanilla extract

6 oz. pkg. semi-sweet chocolate chips

1 pkg. chocolate cake mix (plus ingredients required for cake—see package)

Line muffin pan with paper liner cups. Cream together cream cheese and sugar. Beat in egg, salt, vanilla, and add chocolate chips. Set aside. Prepare cake mix per package instructions. Spoon cake mix into muffin liners then drop a rounded teaspoonful of cream cheese mixture in the center of each cupcake. Bake according to cake mix package directions.

BLUEBERRY DELIGHT

(Serves 16—a great company dessert and family favorite!)

2 c. graham cracker crumbs (26 crackers)

1½ c. sugar (divided portions)

½ c. butter or margarine

4 eggs, beaten

1 tsp. vanilla

2 - 8 oz. pkgs. cream cheese, softened

2 cans blueberry pie filling

whipped cream (sweetened) or Cool Whip

Preheat oven to 350°. Blend together crumbs, ½ c. sugar, and butter. Press this mixture into the bottom of a 9" x 12" dish. To the eggs, add 1 c. sugar and cream cheese and blend well. Spread over graham cracker mixture and bake at 350° for 25 min. Cool. Spread layer of blueberry pie filling and top with layer of whipped cream. Serve cold.

Enough already!

I hope you have found some of my coping hints for your 80s and 90s to be helpful. Thank you for sharing your time with me, and I will close with one final suggestion: Have you ever thought about writing a book of your own? Tell your family story, share some advice, or make up a good tale. I think you will enjoy it, as I have.

May your days be full and strong and rich with blessings.

Your friend,

Bee

At the End of the Day:

A Letter from the Author's Daughters

Recently, Mother was discussing the state of our great nation and the sad reality that the mighty USA has drifted far from the founding concept, "In God We Trust." Mom calls it "slouching toward Gomorrah."

She laments the negative influence of most television, the decline of personal morality and responsibility, "it's-all-about-me-ness," and children who have more rights than respect. She sometimes wonders how much longer she wants to be here.

"Maybe Jesus will come today," said Melinda, the first-born, "and you can go straight to heaven. Just think! You wouldn't have to suffer in dying."

"Well," Mother answered, true to form, "I'm not afraid of dying. I just don't want to be there when it happens."

This is our mom in a nutshell—practical, joking, grounded.

And always ready with another quip: "Besides, I read the book *Left Behind*. When they were taken up, they left their clothes behind. I don't think I want to be flying around heaven in a 93-year-old naked body. At my present weight of 103 (give or take a pound), I'd look like a pregnant skeleton."

Mother fears this writing makes her sound like a saint, and "saint I ain't," she insists. She is determined that her book, which she refers to as a letter, is not about her. "I want to be short on *I, me,* and *us,* and long on helpful hints," she says. Yet as her children, we feel a glimpse into the "I, me, and us" of our family might also provide useful clues about living to the fullest at every age.

Dad was a country boy. The little Wildwood church where he grew up, started in 1854, is still active and serving its purpose. He still remembers the hot day of his confirmation—the windows open wide and cardboard fans flapping. He and the one other confirmand were swatting wasps to keep from being stung during the ceremony. Afterwards, the small congregation gathered under a sprawling, old oak and spread the tables for a potluck dinner. Except for the confirmation, this was how Dad spent Sundays with his family. Every Sunday.

We can imagine mother walking hand-in-hand with her father to church downtown. He stops to move a snail from the sidewalk to safer ground, or he spies some other critter. He's hoping the little thing wasn't injured or in need of help; if it was, it was going to church and then home with them afterward to be tended. Papaw was a healer, or at least he tried to be.

These seeds planted in our parents' youth flourished when they married and started a family of their own. We two sisters were raised in what was at that time an average, comfortable, two-parent home. Our dad worked hard so our mom could be a full-time housewife and mother—a full time job!

We went out as a family, including a two-week road trip every summer. Every Easter, we had a new dress, which mom made, plus new shoes and a spring coat. She made all our clothes and taught us how to do so too.

We had the best birthday parties. Can you imagine letting little children pull taffy in your kitchen and then roll it in powdered sugar?

We worked on projects—often placing high in science fairs. For every talent show, we practiced hard and did well in the days long before everyone started lessons at age three. Melinda's starring number was "I'm Little, Short and Puny but I'm Loud," and Holly's moment in the spotlight was "I'm a Lonely Little Petunia in an Onion Patch," wearing a mother-crafted petunia costume. We were Bluebirds and Campfire Girls. Mom led, and Dad participated. We sang and made music, played cards and dominoes. Life was simpler back then!

But their greatest gift of all was raising us securely in the arms of Christ. Ever heard the expression, "They were there every time the church doors opened"? That was us. Mom taught Sunday School, and Dad held church leadership positions. We sang in the choirs, attended Bible School, performed in the Christmas pageants, and went on mission and pleasure trips with the youth group. They brought us up *in* the church.

We both have among our cherished possessions our "Perfect Attendance" pins from Sunday School. Each year, we joyfully added another little bar to the bottom. Being in church was a priority. Even on vacation, our parents sought out a local church that we could attend.

Even so, we knew faith was not about pins on our collars. It was something we lived—the fabric of our lives. It was really very simple: love God, help others, and do the right thing.

You see, this is how our parents "did" religion. Mother didn't talk about it by evangelizing, but she talked about it constantly in the focus of our lives: mealtime prayers and bedtime prayers, getting ready for church, or vacation Bible School, taking a group of kids caroling at the old folks home at Christmas, or the perpetual piles of rummage gathered in our garage for "Operation Salvage," the drive she started decades before it became common to donate and recycle.

We are reminded of Matthew 25:35-36:

For I was hungry, and you fed me. I was thirsty, and you gave me a drink. I was a stranger, and you invited me into your home. I was naked, and you gave me clothing. I was sick, and you cared for me (NLT).

Every Sunday, at age 93, our parents still take individual servings of whatever they have eaten during the week to a friend who lives alone and isn't well. Likewise, they are ready to meet the needs of a worker in the yard or a complete stranger walking on their street, going out of their way to help if it might be needed. And our mom and dad still open their home to any friend who might need a place to land.

From her work with Operation Salvage 30 odd years ago, it occurred to Mom that no one bought wool skirts. A recycler well before her time, she began cutting the garments apart, down to ripping out and flattening waistbands. From these scraps, she pieced together blankets. Patterns were random, colorful, and sometimes quite pretty. She and her growing group of quilt makers, "Cover Girls" she dubbed them, added layers of other salvaged materials so the blankets would be warmer.

Mom has no idea how many blankets they shipped off to relief agencies (well more than 1000 by our reckoning). She never kept records; that wasn't the point. She did it because good wool was being wasted, and people needed warmth.

Her reward was the thought that somewhere someone was comforted under a blanket she made from skirts nobody wanted. One time she thought she recognized one of her quilts in a news report. It was wrapped over the shoulders of a small boy riding the back of a camel.

Our dad is still the first call for many in need of a ride to the doctor or a run for a prescription. Perhaps this is the continuation of the Ken Lewis Ministry that Mother started years ago. Church members would stand ready, willing, and able to help one another with small tasks not easily managed, perhaps something as simple as changing a light bulb.

Our parents always tithed. We remember Mom saying that sometimes when things were really tight, she would write the check to the church on the first then hold it until the end of the month. Every single time, she was able to go ahead and give it.

Melinda recently attended worship with our parents at their church. The groundskeeping team was listed in the bulletin, and lo and behold, Charlie Oldfield was listed as its head. Mother says that at 93 he ought to be allowed to retire from lawn mowing duty. Where are the younger men? But Dad replies with a signature chuckle, "Finally I made it to the top! Now I can boss the younger guys around."

Could it be that hard work, a good sense of humor, and a focus on what really matters are what keep them going?

These days, our folks are comfortable. Dad often says he never dreamed when growing up that he would be so blessed.

Mom and Dad don't wear Christianity on their sleeves; they wear it like skin. We can't help but wonder if this is the real key to living life to one's fullest at whatever age.

—*Melinda O'Neal and Holly Hughes*